Table of Contents

INTRODUCTION 4

FOOD POISONING SYMPTOMS.. 5

Causes of food poisoning 6

Bacteria... 7

Parasites 8

Trichinella 9

Viruses 9

Food poisoning treatments 10

Off-Label Drug Use 14

What to eat and drink when you have food poisoning..... 15

What to avoid 16

How food poisoning is diagnosed............................ 17

Risk factors for food poisoning............................... 17

How to prevent food poisoning............................... 19

10 SIGNS AND SYMPTOMS OF FOOD POISONING..................... 21

IS FOOD POISONING CONTAGIOUS? 27

Types of food poisoning 28

How to prevent the spread of food poisoning 32

What is the outlook for food poisoning?......................... 34

TOP 9 FOODS MOST LIKELY TO CAUSE FOOD POISONING........ 41

How to Reduce Your Risk of Food Poisoning......................... 53

WHAT SUPPORTIVE THERAPIES TREAT FOOD POISONING? 56

When should you consult with a doctor or other healthcare
professional? 60

WHY COOKING CHICKEN TO 165 DEGREES IS CRITICAL FOR
ENSURING SAFETY, PREVENTING ILLNESS................................. 66

CONCLUSION 69

INTRODUCTION

Food poisoning usually isn't life threatening. It can be uncomfortable, but most people recover completely within a few days even without treatment. Foodborne illness, more commonly referred to as food poisoning, is the result of eating contaminated, spoiled, or toxic food. The most common symptoms of food poisoning include nausea, vomiting, and diarrhea. Although it's quite uncomfortable, food poisoning isn't unusual. According to the Centers for Disease Control and Prevention (CDC)Trusted Source, 48 million people in the United States (or around 1 out of 7) contract some form of food poisoning every year. Of those 48 million people, 128,000 are hospitalized.

FOOD POISONING SYMPTOMS

If you have food poisoning, chances are it won't go undetected. Symptoms can vary depending on the source of the infection. Common cases of food poisoning will typically include a few of the following symptoms:

- abdominal cramps

- diarrhea

- nausea

- vomiting

- loss of appetite

- mild fever

- weakness

- headache

Symptoms of potentially life threatening food poisoning include:

diarrhea that lasts for more than 3 days

a fever higher than 102°F (38.9°C)

difficulty seeing or speaking

symptoms of severe dehydration, which may include dry mouth, passing little to no urine, and difficulty keeping fluids down bloody urine

If you experience any of these symptoms, contact a doctor or seek medical treatment immediately.

Causes of food poisoning

Most food poisoning can be traced to one of three major causes: bacteria, parasites, or viruses. These pathogens can be found on almost all of the food humans eat. However, heat from cooking usually kills pathogens on food before it reaches our plate. Foods eaten raw are common sources of food poisoning because they don't go through the cooking process.

Occasionally, food will come in contact with the organisms in fecal matter or vomit. This is most likely to occur when an ill person prepares food and doesn't wash their hands before cooking. Meat, eggs, and dairy products are frequently contaminated. Water may also be contaminated with organisms that cause illness.

Bacteria
Bacteria are by far the most common cause of food poisoning. Bacterial causes of food poisoning include:

E. coli, in particular Shiga toxin-producing E. coli (STEC)

Listeria monocytogenes

Salmonella

Campylobacter

Clostridium botulinum

Staphylococcus aureus

Shigella

Vibrio vulnificus

When thinking of dangerous bacteria, names such as E. coli and Salmonella come to mind for good reason. Salmonella is the biggest bacterial causeTrusted Source of food poisoning cases in the United States. According to the CDCTrusted Source, an estimated 1,350,000 cases of food poisoning, including 26,500 hospitalizations, can be traced to salmonella infection each year.

Campylobacter and C. botulinum are two lesser-known and potentially lethal bacteria that can lurk in our food.

Parasites
Food poisoning caused by parasites isn't as common as food poisoning caused by bacteria, but parasites that spread through food are still very dangerous. They include:

Toxoplasma gondii

Giardia lamblia

various tapeworms, such as:

Taenia saginata (beef tapeworm)

Taenia solium (pork tapeworm)

Diphyllobothrium latum (fish tapeworm)

Cryptosporidium

Ascaris lumbricoides, a type of roundworm

flukes (flatworms), such as Opisthorchiidae (liver fluke) and Paragonimus (lung fluke)

pinworms, or Enterobiasis

Trichinella
According to the CDC, toxoplasmosis is a leading cause of death attributed to food poisoning in the United States. Toxoplasma gondii is also found in cat litter boxes. Parasites can live in your digestive tract and go undetected for years. People with weakened immune systems and pregnant people are at risk of more serious side effects if certain parasites take up residence in their intestines.

Viruses
Food poisoning can also be caused by a virus, such as:

norovirus, which is sometimes known as Norwalk virus

rotavirus

astrovirus

sapovirus

hepatitis A virus

The norovirus causes 19 to 21 million casesTrusted Source of vomiting and diarrhea in the United States each year. In rare cases, it can be fatal. Other viruses bring on similar symptoms, but they're less common. The virus that causes the liver condition hepatitis A can also be transmitted through food.

Food poisoning treatments

Food poisoning can usually be treated at home. Here are some ways you can help treat food poisoning:

Stay hydrated

If you have food poisoning, it's crucial to remain properly hydrated. Sports drinks high in electrolytes can be helpful. Fruit juice and coconut water can restore carbohydrates and help with fatigue. Avoid caffeine, which may irritate the digestive tract. Decaffeinated teas with soothing herbs such as chamomile, peppermint, and dandelion may help calm an upset stomach.

Take over-the-counter (OTC) medications

Over-the-counter (OTC) medications such as loperamide (Imodium) and Pepto-Bismol can help you manage diarrhea and suppress nausea. However, you should check with a doctor before using these medications, as the body uses vomiting and diarrhea to rid the system of the toxin. Also, using these medications could mask the severity of the illness and cause you to delay seeking expert treatment. Pyrantel pamoate (Reese's Pinworm Medicine) is a common remedy for pinworms.

Take prescription medications

Although many cases of food poisoning clear up on their own, some people can benefit from prescription medications, depending on the pathogen responsible for their illness. Prescription medications may benefit people who are older, immunocompromised, or pregnant. For pregnant people, antibiotic treatment helps prevent an infection from being transmitted to the unborn baby. If you require prescription medications, your doctor may recommend one of these regimens for the following causes of illness:

A. lumbricoides: the antiparasitic medications albendazole (Albenza) or mebendazole (Enverm)

Campylobacter: the antibiotic azithromycin (Zithromax)

Cryptosporidium: the antiparasitic medication nitazoxanide (Alinia), which is used to treat diarrhea

D. latum (fish tapeworm): the antiparasitic medication praziquantel (Biltricide)

Enterobiasis (pinworms): albendazole (Albenza) or mebendazole (Enverm)

G. lamblia:

nitazoxanide (Alinia)

the antibiotics metronidazole (Flagyl), paromomycin, quinacrine, or furazolidone

tinidazole (Tindamax), which is an antibiotic and antiparasitic medication

L. monocytogenes: the antibiotic ampicillin

Opisthorchiidae (liver fluke): praziquantel (Biltricide) or albendazole (Albenza)

Paragonimus (lung fluke): praziquantel (Biltricide) or the antiparasitic medication triclabendazole (Egaten)

Shigella: the antibiotics azithromycin (Zithromax) or ciprofloxacin (Cipro)

T. saginata (beef tapeworm): praziquantel (Biltricide) or albendazole (Albenza), which are off-label treatments for T. saginata

T. solium (pork tapeworm): praziquantel (Biltricide) or albendazole (Albenza), which are off-label treatments for T. solium

T. gondii:

a combination of the antiparasitic medication pyrimethamine (Daraprim) and an antibiotic such as sulfadiazine

the antibiotic spiramycin, as a standalone medication

Trichinella: albendazole (Albenza) or mebendazole (Enverm)

Off-Label Drug Use

Off-label drug use means a drug that's approved by the Food and Drug Administration (FDA) for one purpose is used for a different purpose that hasn't yet been approved. However, a doctor can still use the drug for that purpose. This is because the FDA regulates the testing and approval of drugs but not how doctors use drugs to treat their patients. So your doctor can prescribe a drug however they think is best for your care.

Receive an antitoxin

An infection with C. botulinum is considered a medical emergency. Seek medical care as soon as you can. If you have a case of C. botulinum, a doctor will administer an antitoxin. Babies will receive a special antitoxin called BabyBIG (botulism immune globulin).

Rest

It's also important for those with food poisoning to get plenty of rest. If your case is severe

In severe cases of food poisoning, you may require hydration with intravenous (IV) fluid at a hospital. In the very worst cases of food poisoning, a longer hospital stay may be required while you recover. People with severe cases of C. botulinum, which are rare, may even require mechanical ventilation.

What to eat and drink when you have food poisoning

It's best to gradually hold off on solid foods until diarrhea and vomiting have passed. Instead, ease back into your regular diet by eating or drinking simple-to-digest items that are bland and low in fat, such as:

saltine crackers

toast

gelatin

bananas

rice

oatmeal

bland potatoes

boiled vegetables

chicken broth

soda without caffeine, such as ginger ale or root beer

diluted fruit juices

sports drinks

What to avoid
To prevent your stomach from getting more upset, try to avoid the following harder-to-digest foods, even if you think you feel better:

dairy products, especially milk and cheeses

fatty foods

fried foods

highly seasoned foods

foods that are high in sugar

spicy foods

Also avoid:

caffeine

alcohol

nicotine

How food poisoning is diagnosed

A doctor may be able to diagnose the type of food poisoning based on your symptoms. In severe cases, blood tests, stool tests, and tests on food that you've eaten may be conducted to determine what's responsible for the food poisoning. A doctor may also use a urine test to evaluate whether you are dehydrated as a result of food poisoning.

Risk factors for food poisoning

Anyone can come down with food poisoning. Statistically speaking, nearly everyone will come down with food poisoning at least once in their lives. There are some populations that are more at risk than others. These include:

Immunocompromised people. Anyone with a suppressed immune system or an autoimmune disease may have a greater risk of infection and complications resulting from food poisoning.

Pregnant people. Pregnant people are more at risk because their bodies are coping with changes to their metabolism and circulatory system during pregnancy.

Older adults. Adults who are 65 years or older also face a greater risk of contracting food poisoning. This is because their immune systems may not respond quickly to infectious organisms.

Young children. Children under 5 years old are also considered an at-risk population because their immune systems aren't as developed as those of adults. Young children are more easily affected by dehydration from vomiting and diarrhea.

How to prevent food poisoning

The best way to prevent food poisoning is to handle your food safely and avoid any food that may be unsafe. Some foods are more likely to cause food poisoning because of the way they're produced and prepared. Infectious agents that are killed during cooking may be present in certain foods, such as:

meat

poultry

eggs

shellfish

Food poisoning can occur if these foods are eaten in their raw form, not cooked properly, or if hands and surfaces aren't cleaned after contact. Other foods that are likely to cause food poisoning include:

sushi and other fish products that are served raw or undercooked deli meats and hot dogs that aren't heated or cooked

ground beef, which may contain meat from several animals

unpasteurized milk, cheese, and juice

raw, unwashed fruits and vegetables

To try to avoid food poisoning, take these steps:

Always wash your hands before cooking or eating food.

Make sure your food is properly sealed and stored.

Thoroughly cook meat and eggs.

Sanitize anything that comes in contact with raw products before using it to prepare other foods.

Make sure to always wash fruits and vegetables before serving them.

Outlook for food poisoning

It's extremely rare for food poisoning to be life threatening. While having food poisoning is quite uncomfortable, the good news is that most people recover completely within a few days, even without treatment.

10 SIGNS AND SYMPTOMS OF FOOD POISONING

1. Abdominal pain and cramps

Abdominal pain caused by food poisoning is felt around the trunk of your body. Harmful toxins irritate your stomach lining, causing cramping that is worsened when your abdominal muscles work to get rid of the organisms. However, abdominal pain and cramps may be caused by other things than food poisoning. Because of this, these symptoms alone may not be a sign of food poisoning. Furthermore, not all cases of food poisoning will result in abdominal pain or cramps.Abdominal pain and cramps can indicate inflammation in your stomach and intestines. Cramping may also occur as your body tries to eliminate harmful organisms.

2. Diarrhea

Diarrhea is watery and loose stools occurring three or more times in a 24-hour period, and it's often caused by food poisoning. It's usually accompanied by an urgent feeling for the bathroom and bloating/abdominal cramps. Diarrhea occurs as inflammation makes your bowel less effective at reabsorbing the water and other fluids it secretes during digestion. This means it raises your chance of becoming dehydrated. Make sure to drink fluids such as water or broth and check that urine color is light yellow to clear. Diarrhea consists of three or more loose, watery stools in 24 hours. The biggest health risk of diarrhea is dehydration, so it's important to drink enough fluids.

3. Headaches

Headaches are extremely common Stress, alcohol, dehydration, and fatigue can all be causes. Food poisoning may also lead to a headache, as it can cause both fatigue and dehydration. Vomiting and diarrhea also increase your chance of dehydration-related headaches. You may get a headache when you have food poisoning, especially if you become dehydrated.

4. Vomiting

Vomiting is a natural response to food poisoning. It happens when your body tries to expel harmful organisms or toxins. Some experience projectile vomiting that subsides quickly, while others vomit intermittently for several days. If you can't keep fluids down, seek medical help to avoid dehydration. Many people with food poisoning vomit. It's a protective mechanism that helps your body remove harmful organisms you have eaten.

5. Generally feeling sick

Food poisoning often causes loss of appetite and fatigue as your immune system responds to the infection. Your body releases chemical messengers called cytokines, which have many different roles. These include regulating your body's immune response and signaling to the brain to trigger the symptoms we generally associate with illness. This collection of symptoms can result in what is sometimes called "sickness behavior," as you withdraw from social interactions, rest and stop eating. It's a sign that your body is diverting its attention from other body processes like digestion to prioritize fighting an infection. Cytokines are chemical messengers that are important in regulating your immune response. Their presence also causes some of the typical symptoms of illness, such as loss of appetite.

6. Fever

A fever is when your body temperature rises above 97.6–99.6°F (36–37°C). Fevers occur as part of your body's natural defense against infection. Fever-producing substances called pyrogens are released by your immune system or by the invading bacteria. They trigger a rise in temperature by making your brain think you're colder than you really are. This helps boost the activity of white blood cells as they fight the infection Fever is a common symptom of illness. It helps fight infection by making your body too hot, which helps your immune system fight infection.

7. Chills

Chills can occur as your body shivers to raise your temperature. These shivers result from your muscles rapidly contracting and relaxing, which generates heat. They often accompany a fever, as pyrogens trick your body into thinking it's cold and need to warm up. A fever can occur with many different illnesses, including food poisoning, making chills one of its common symptoms. Chills often accompany a fever, which can occur in cases of food poisoning. Thinking it's too cold, your body shivers in an attempt to warm up.

8. Weakness and fatigue

Feeling weak or tired can be a symptom of food poisoning, partly due to the release of chemical messengers called cytokines. These symptoms are also signs of sickness behavior, which helps you rest and recover. If you experience this, it is best to listen to your body and rest. Weakness and fatigue are common side effects of food poisoning caused by chemical messengers called cytokines released by your body when you are sick.

9. Nausea

Nausea is how you feel when you're about to vomit. It can be caused by things like food poisoning, migraine, or motion sickness (25Trusted Source).

In case of an infection, it is a warning sign that you may have eaten something harmful. If you feel nauseous, you might want to try some of these natural remedies to help relieve your symptoms. Nausea is the debilitating feeling of being queasy before you are sick. It serves as a warning signal of food poisoning.

10. Muscle aches

When you get an infection, like food poisoning, you can get muscle pain. This happens because your body releases histamine to widen your blood vessels and allow your white blood cells to fight the infection. Cytokines and other substances involved in the immune response can reach other parts of your body, triggering pain receptors and causing aching. An infection like food poisoning can make your body ache due to inflammation caused by the immune system's response.

To prevent food poisoning, it's a good idea to practice good hygiene in the kitchen and wash your hands. Most cases of food poisoning are not serious and will subside on their own. If symptoms linger, it's best to rest, stay hydrated, and see a doctor if symptoms don't improve in a few days.

IS FOOD POISONING CONTAGIOUS?

Food poisoning caused by some bacteria, viruses, or parasites can be contagious. Cases caused by chemicals or toxins can't be spread to others. Food poisoning, also called foodborne illness, is caused by eating or drinking contaminated food or drinks. Symptoms of food poisoning vary but can include nausea, vomiting, diarrhea, and abdominal cramps. Some people also develop a fever. Of an estimated 48 million people who become sick from foodborne illnesses each year in the United States, 3,000 will die, according to the Centers for Disease Control and Prevention (CDC).

Symptoms can develop within hours or days of eating contaminated food. Food poisoning that is caused by certain bacteria, viruses, or parasites is contagious. So, if you or your child has symptoms of food poisoning, take steps to protect yourself and to prevent the spread of the illness. Sometimes, food poisoning is the result of chemicals or toxins found in the food. This type of food poisoning isn't considered to be an infection, so it isn't contagious and doesn't spread from person to person.

Types of food poisoning

There are over 250 different types of foodborne illnesses. Most of these illnesses are caused by one of the following.

1. Bacteria

Bacteria — which are tiny organisms — can get into the gastrointestinal (GI) tract through contaminated food and bring on symptoms like nausea, vomiting, diarrhea, and abdominal pain. Bacteria can contaminate food in a number of ways:

You may purchase food that's already spoiled or contaminated with bacteria.

Your food may become contaminated at some point during storage or preparation.

This can happen if you don't wash your hands before preparing or handling food. It can also happen when food comes in contact with a surface contaminated with bacteria.

Improper storage of food, such as keeping food at room temperature or outdoors for too long, can also cause bacteria to grow and multiply rapidly.

It's important to refrigerate or freeze food after cooking. Don't eat food that's been left sitting out for too long. Keep in mind that contaminated food may taste and smell normal. Bacteria that can cause food poisoning include:

Salmonella

Shigella

E. coli (some strains, including E. coli O157:H7)

Listeria

Campylobacter jejuni

Staphylococcus aureus (staph)

2. Viruses

Food poisoning caused by viruses can also pass from person to person. A common foodborne virus is norovirus, which causes inflammation in the stomach and intestines. Hepatitis A is another foodborne illness from a virus. This highly contagious acute liver infection causes inflammation of the liver. Hepatitis A virus can be found in the stool and blood of people who are infected. If you don't wash your hands after using the bathroom, it's possible to pass the virus to others through handshakes and other physical contact. You may also spread the virus to others if you prepare food or drinks with contaminated hands.

Contagious foodborne viruses also spread through indirect contact. Throughout the course of a day, you may touch several surfaces with contaminated hands. These include light switches, counters, phones, and door handles. Anyone who touches these surfaces may become ill if they put their hands near their mouth. Bacteria and viruses can live outside the body on hard surfaces for hours, and sometimes days. Salmonella and campylobacter can live on surfaces for up to four hours, whereas the norovirus can survive on surfaces for weeks.

3. Parasites

Parasites that can cause food poisoning include:

Giardia duodenalis (formerly known as G. lamblia)

Cryptosporidium parvum

Cyclospora cayetanensis

Toxoplasma gondii

Trichinella spiralis

Taenia saginata

Taenia solium

Parasites are organisms that range in size. Some are microscopic, but others, such as parasite worms, may be visible to the naked eye. These organisms live in or on other organisms (called a host) and receive nutrients from this host. When present, these organisms are found usually in the stool of humans and animals. They can transfer into your body when you eat contaminated food, drink contaminated water, or put anything in your mouth that's come in contact with the feces of an infected person or animal.nYou can spread this type of food poisoning through physical contact or by preparing food with contaminated hands.

How to prevent the spread of food poisoning

Anyone can get food poisoning, but there are ways to prevent its spread once you've been infected. Preventing the spread of contagious foodborne illnesses is important because complications can arise. Since food poisoning can cause vomiting and diarrhea, there's the risk of dehydration. In severe cases of dehydration, hospitalization is required to replace lost fluids. Dehydration can be particularly dangerous for infants, elderly people, and people who have a weak immune system. Here are a few tips to prevent the spread of food poisoning once you're already sick.

Bacteria

Stay home from school or work until symptoms disappear

Wash your hands with warm, soapy water after going to the bathroom and after coming in contact with animal or human feces.

Don't prepare or handle food or drinks until symptoms disappear and you feel better.

Teach children how to properly wash their hands. According to the CDC, proper hand washingTrusted Source should take about 20 seconds, the same length of time it takes to sing the "Happy Birthday" song twice.

Disinfect commonly touched surfaces in the home — light switches, door knobs, countertops, remote controls, etc.

Clean the bathroom toilet after each use, using disinfecting wipes or a disinfectant spray on the seat and handle.

Virus

Stay home from school and work until symptoms disappear and avoid travel.

Wash your hands with warm, soapy water after using the bathroom and after coming in contact with human or animal feces.

Don't prepare or handle food or drinks until symptoms disappear and you feel better.

Disinfect surfaces around the house.

Wear gloves when cleaning up the vomit or diarrhea of an infected person.

Parasite

Wash hands with warm, soapy water after going to the bathroom and after coming in contact with human or animal feces

Don't prepare or handle food or drinks until symptoms disappear and you feel better.

Practice safe sex. Some parasites (Giardia) can spread through unprotected oral-anal sex.

What is the outlook for food poisoning?
Food poisoning can cause a variety of uncomfortable symptoms such as diarrhea, vomiting, stomach pain, and a fever. However, symptoms typically resolve on their own within hours to days and don't usually require a doctor. Getting plenty of rest and drinking fluids can help you feel better. Even though you may not feel like eating, your body needs energy, so it's important to nibble on bland foods like crackers, toast, and rice.

Fluids (water, juice, decaffeinated teas) are also vital to avoid dehydration. If you have symptoms of dehydration, go to the hospital immediately. Signs include extreme thirst, infrequent urination, dark-colored urine, fatigue, and dizziness. In children, symptoms of dehydration include a dry tongue, no wet diapers for three hours, weakness, irritability, and crying without tears.

Salmonella Food Poisoning

Certain bacteria in the group Salmonella cause salmonella food poisoning. These bacteria live in the intestines of humans and animals. Human infection results when food or water that has been contaminated with infected feces is ingested. A gastrointestinal salmonella infection usually affects the small intestine. It is also called salmonella enterocolitis or enteric salmonellosis. It's one of the most common types of food poisoning.

Around 19,000 people are hospitalized with salmonella food poisoning every year in the United States. It's most common in people under 20 years old. It's also more likely to occur in the summer months because the Salmonella bacterium grows better in warm weather.

What causes salmonella food poisoning?

Eating food or drinking any liquid contaminated with certain species of Salmonella bacteria causes salmonella food poisoning. People are usually infected by eating raw foods or prepared foods that have been handled by others. Salmonella is often spread when people don't wash (or improperly wash) their hands after using the toilet. It can also be spread by handling pets, especially reptiles and birds. Thorough cooking or pasteurization kills Salmonella bacteria. You're at risk when you consume raw, undercooked, or unpasteurized items. Salmonella food poisoning is commonly caused by:

undercooked chicken, turkey, or other poultry

undercooked eggs

unpasteurized milk or juice

contaminated raw fruits, vegetables, or nuts

A number of factors can increase your risk of salmonella infection, including:

having family members with salmonellafood poisoning

having a pet reptile or bird (they can carry Salmonella)

living in group housing such as dorms or nursing homes, where you're regularly exposed to many people and food preparation by others

traveling to developing countries where sanitation is poor and hygienic standards are substandard. If you have a weakened immune system, you're more likely than others to become infected with Salmonella.

Recognizing the symptoms of salmonella food poisoning

The symptoms of salmonella food poisoning often come on quickly, usually within 8 to 72 hours after consuming contaminated food or water. Symptoms may be aggressive and can last for up to 48 hours. Typical symptoms during this acute stage include:

abdominal pain, cramping, or tenderness

chills

diarrhea

fever

muscle pain

nausea

vomiting

signs of dehydration (such as decreased or dark-colored urine, dry mouth, and low energy)

bloody stool

Dehydration caused by diarrhea is a serious concern, especially in children and infants. The very young can become severely dehydrated in just one day. This can lead to death.

Diagnosing salmonella food poisoning

To diagnose salmonella food poisoning, your doctor will do a physical examination. They may check if your abdomen is tender. They may look for a rash with small pink dots on your skin. If these dots are accompanied by a high fever, they may indicate a serious form of salmonella infection called typhoid fever. Your doctor may also do a blood test or stool culture. This is to look for actual evidence and samples of Salmonella bacteria in your body.

Treating salmonella food poisoning

The main treatment for salmonella food poisoning is replacing fluids and electrolytes that you lose when you have diarrhea. Adults should drink water or suck on ice cubes. Your pediatrician may suggest rehydration drinks such as Pedialyte for children.

In addition, modify your diet to include only easily digestible foods. Bananas, rice, applesauce, and toast are good options. You should avoid dairy products and get plenty of rest. This allows your body to fight the infection. If nausea prevents you from drinking liquids, you may need to see your doctor and receive intravenous (IV) fluids. Young children may also need IV fluids.

Typically, antibiotics and medication to stop your diarrhea aren't recommended. These treatments can prolong the "carrier state" and the infection, respectively. The "carrier state" is the period of time during and after the infection when you can transmit the infection to another person. You should consult with your doctor about medications for symptom management. In severe or life-threatening cases, your doctor may prescribe antibiotics.

Preventing salmonella food poisoning

To help prevent salmonella food poisoning:

Handle food properly. Cook foods to recommended internal temperatures, and refrigerate leftovers promptly.

Clean counters before and after preparing high-risk foods.

Wash your hands thoroughly (especially when handling eggs or poultry).

Use separate utensils for raw and cooked items.

Keep foods refrigerated before cooking.

If you own a reptile or bird, wear gloves or wash your hands thoroughly after handling.

People who have salmonella and work in the food service industry should not return to work until they haven't had diarrhea for at least 48 hours.

Salmonella food poisoning outlook

For healthy people, symptoms should go away within two to seven days. However, the bacteria can stay in the body longer. This means that even if you aren't experiencing symptoms, you can still infect other people with Salmonella bacteria.

TOP 9 FOODS MOST LIKELY TO CAUSE FOOD POISONING

Improper food storage, preparation, and hygiene can lead to food poisoning. Some foods to pay special attention to while preparing that commonly cause food poisoning include meat products, leafy greens, and rice. Food poisoning happens when people consume food that is contaminated with harmful bacteria, parasites, viruses or toxins.

Also known as foodborne illness, it can cause a range of symptoms, most commonly stomach cramps, diarrhea, vomiting, nausea and loss of appetite. Pregnant women, young children, the elderly and people with chronic illnesses have a greater risk of becoming ill with food poisoning.Certain foods are more likely to cause food poisoning than others, especially if they are improperly stored, prepared or cooked.Here are the top 9 foods that are most likely to cause food poisoning.

1. Poultry

Raw and undercooked poultry such as chicken, duck and turkey has a high risk of causing food poisoning. This is mainly due to two types of bacteria, Campylobacter and Salmonella, which are commonly found in the guts and feathers of these birds. These bacteria often contaminate fresh poultry meat during the slaughtering process, and they can survive up until cooking kills them. In fact, research from the UK, US and Ireland found that 41–84% of raw chicken sold in supermarkets was contaminated with

Campylobacter bacteria and 4–5% was contaminated with Salmonella (3Trusted Source, 4Trusted Source, 5Trusted Source).

The rates of Campylobacter contamination were slightly lower in raw turkey meat, ranging from 14–56%, while the contamination rate for raw duck meat was 36%. The good news is that although these harmful bacteria can live on raw poultry, they're completely eliminated when meat is cooked thoroughly. To reduce your risk, ensure poultry meat is cooked through completely, do not wash raw meat and ensure that raw meat does not come in contact with utensils, kitchen surfaces, chopping boards and other foods, since this can result in cross-contamination. Raw and undercooked poultry is a common source of food poisoning. To reduce your risk, thoroughly cook chicken, duck and turkey meat. This will eliminate any harmful bacteria present.

2. Vegetables and Leafy Greens

Vegetables and leafy greens are a common source of food poisoning, especially when eaten raw. In fact, fruits and vegetables have caused a number food poisoning outbreaks, particularly lettuce, spinach, cabbage, celery and tomatoes. Vegetables and leafy greens can become contaminated with harmful bacteria, such as E. coli, Salmonella and Listeria. This can occur across various stages of the supply chain. Contamination can occur from unclean water and dirty runoff, which can leach into the soil that fruits and vegetables are grown in (11Trusted Source).

It can also occur from dirty processing equipment and unhygienic food preparation practices. Leafy greens are especially risky because they are often consumed raw. In fact, between 1973 and 2012, 85% of the food poisoning outbreaks in the US that were caused by leafy greens such as cabbage, kale, lettuce and spinach were traced back to food prepared in a restaurant or catering facility. To minimize your risk, always wash salad leaves thoroughly before eating. Do not purchase bags of salad mix that contain spoiled, mushy leaves and avoid pre-prepared salads that have been left to sit at room temperature.

Vegetables and leafy greens can often carry harmful bacteria such as E. coli, Salmonella and Listeria. To reduce your risk, always wash vegetables and salad leaves and only purchase prepackaged salads that have been refrigerated.

3. Fish and Shellfish

Fish and shellfish are a common source of food poisoning. Fish that has not been stored at the correct temperature has a high risk of being contaminated with histamine, a toxin produced by bacteria in fish. Histamine is not destroyed by normal cooking temperatures and results in a type of food poisoning known as scombroid poisoning. It causes a range of symptoms including nausea, wheezing and swelling of the face and tongue. Another type of food poisoning caused by contaminated fish is ciguatera fish poisoning (CFP). This occurs due to a toxin called ciguatoxin, which is mostly found in warm, tropical waters.

At least 10,000–50,000 people who live in or visit tropical areas get CFP each year, according to estimates. Like histamine, it is not destroyed by normal cooking temperatures and therefore the harmful toxins are present after cooking. Shellfish such as clams, mussels, oysters and scallops also carry a risk of food poisoning. Algae that are consumed by shellfish produce many toxins, and these can build up in the flesh of shellfish, posing danger to humans when they consume the shellfish. Store-bought shellfish are usually safe to eat. However, shellfish caught from unmonitored areas may be unsafe due to contamination from sewage, stormwater drains and septic tanks.

To reduce your risk, purchase store-bought seafood and ensure you keep it chilled and refrigerated before cooking. Make sure fish is cooked through, and cook clams, mussels and oysters till the shells open. Throw away the shells that don't open. Fish and shellfish are a common source of food poisoning due to the presence of histamine and toxins. To reduce your risk, stick with store-bought seafood and keep it chilled before use.

4. Rice

Rice is one of the oldest cereal grains and a staple food for more than half the world's population. However, it is a high-risk food when it comes to food poisoning. Uncooked rice can be contaminated with spores of Bacillus cereus, a bacterium that produces toxins that cause food poisoning. These spores can live in dry conditions. For example, they can survive in a package of uncooked rice in your pantry. They can also survive the cooking process. If cooked rice is left standing at room temperature, these spores grow into bacteria that thrive and multiply in the warm, moist environment. The longer rice is left standing at room temperature, the more likely it will be unsafe to eat. To reduce your risk, serve rice as soon as it has been cooked and refrigerate leftover rice as quickly as possible after cooking. When reheating cooked rice, make sure it is steaming hot all the way through. Rice is a high-risk food due to Bacillus cereus. Spores of this bacterium can live in uncooked rice, and can grow and multiply once rice is cooked. To reduce your risk, eat rice as soon as it is cooked and refrigerate leftovers immediately.

5. Deli Meats

Deli meats including ham, bacon, salami and hot dogs can be a source of food poisoning. They can become contaminated with harmful bacteria including Listeria and Staphylococcus aureus at several stages during processing and manufacturing. Contamination can occur directly through contact with contaminated raw meat or by poor hygiene by deli staff, poor cleaning practices and cross-contamination from unclean equipment such as slicer blades. The reported rates of Listeria in sliced beef, turkey, chicken, ham and paté range from 0–6%.

Of all the deaths caused by Listeria-contaminated deli meats, 83% were caused by deli meat sliced and packaged at deli counters, while 17% were caused by pre-packaged deli meat products. It is important to note that all meat carries a risk of food poisoning if it is not cooked or stored properly.

Hotdogs, minced meat, sausages and bacon should be cooked thoroughly and should be consumed immediately after being cooked. Sliced lunch meats should be stored in the refrigerator until they are ready to be eaten. Deli meats including ham, salami and hot dogs can be contaminated with bacteria that cause food poisoning. It is important to store deli meats in the refrigerator and cook meat thoroughly before eating.

6. Unpasteurized Dairy

Pasteurization is the process of heating a liquid or food to kill harmful microorganisms. Food manufacturers pasteurize dairy products including milk and cheese to make them safe to consume. Pasteurization kills harmful bacteria and parasites such as Brucella, Campylobacter, Cryptosporidium, E. coli, Listeria and Salmonella. In fact, sales of unpasteurized milk and milk products are illegal in 20 US states. Between 1993 and 2006, there were more than 1,500 cases of food poisoning, 202 hospitalizations and two deaths in the US resulting from drinking milk or eating cheese made with unpasteurized milk (28Trusted Source).

What's more, unpasteurized milk is at least 150 times more likely to cause food poisoning and 13 times more likely to result in hospitalization than pasteurized dairy products. To minimize your risk of food poisoning from unpasteurized dairy, purchase pasteurized products only. Store all dairy at or under 40°F (5°C) and throw out dairy that is past its use-by date. Pasteurization involves heating foods and liquids to kill harmful microorganisms such as bacteria. Unpasteurized dairy has been associated with a high risk of food poisoning.

7. Eggs

While eggs are incredibly nutritious and versatile, they can also be a source of food poisoning when they're consumed raw or undercooked. This is because eggs can carry Salmonella bacteria, which can contaminate both the eggshell and the inside of the egg. In the 1970s and 1980s, contaminated eggs were a major source of Salmonella poisoning in the US. The good news is that since 1990, improvements have been made in egg processing and production, which has led to fewer Salmonella outbreaks. In spite of this, each year Salmonella-contaminated eggs cause about 79,000 cases of food poisoning and 30 deaths, according to the US Food and Drug Administration (FDA). To reduce your risk, do not consume eggs with a cracked or dirty shell. Where possible, choose pasteurized eggs in recipes that call for raw or lightly cooked eggs. Raw and undercooked eggs can carry Salmonella bacteria. Choose pasteurized eggs when possible and avoid eggs that have cracked or dirty shells.

8. Fruit

A number of fruit products including berries, melons and pre-prepared fruit salads have been linked to food poisoning outbreaks. Fruits grown on the ground such as cantaloupe (rockmelon), watermelon and honeydew melon have a high risk of causing food poisoning due to Listeria bacteria, which can grow on the rind and spread to the flesh. Between 1973 and 2011, there were 34 reported outbreaks of food poisoning associated with melons in the US. This resulted in 3,602 reported cases of illness, 322 hospitalizations and 46 deaths.

Cantaloupes accounted for 56% of the outbreaks, watermelons accounted for 38% and honeydew melons accounted for 6%. Cantaloupe is a particularly high-risk fruit due to its rough, netted skin, which provides protection for Listeria and other bacteria. This makes it difficult to completely remove bacteria, even with cleaning.

Fresh and frozen berries including raspberries, blackberries, strawberries and blueberries are also a common source of food poisoning due to harmful viruses and bacteria, particularly the hepatitis A virus. The main causes of berry contamination include being grown in contaminated water, poor hygiene practices of berry pickers and cross-contamination with infected berries during processing.

Washing fruit before you eat it can reduce the risks, as can cooking it. If you're eating melon, make sure to wash the rind. Eat fruit as soon as it's cut or place it in the fridge. Avoid pre-packaged fruit salads that have not been chilled or stored in a fridge. Fruits carry a high risk of food poisoning, particularly melon and berries. Always wash fruit before eating and eat freshly cut fruit right away or store it in the fridge.

9. Sprouts

Raw sprouts of any kind, including alfalfa, sunflower, mung bean and clover sprouts, are considered to have a high risk of causing food poisoning. This is mainly due to the presence of bacteria including Salmonella, E. coli and Listeria. Seeds require warm, moist and nutrient-rich conditions for the sprouts to grow. These conditions are ideal for the rapid growth of bacteria. From 1998 to 2010, 33 outbreaks from seed and bean sprouts were documented in the US, and were reported to have affected 1,330 people

In 2014, beansprouts contaminated with Salmonella bacteria caused food poisoning in 115 people, a quarter of whom were hospitalized. The FDA advises that pregnant women avoid consuming any type of raw sprouts. This is because pregnant women are particularly vulnerable to the effects of harmful bacteria. Fortunately, cooking sprouts helps kill any harmful microorganisms and reduces the risk of food poisoning. Sprouts grow in moist, warm conditions and are an ideal environment for the growth of bacteria. Cooking sprouts can help reduce the risk of food poisoning.

How to Reduce Your Risk of Food Poisoning

Here are some simple tips to help minimize your risk of food poisoning:

Practice good hygiene: Wash your hands with soap and hot water before preparing food. Always wash your hands right after touching raw meat and poultry.

Avoid washing raw meat and poultry: This does not kill the bacteria — it only spreads it to other foods, cooking utensils and kitchen surfaces.

Avoid cross-contamination: Use separate chopping boards and knives, especially for raw meat and poultry.

Don't ignore the use-by date: For health and safety reasons, foods should not be eaten after their use-by date. Check use-by dates on your food regularly and throw it out once they've passed, even if the food looks and smells ok.

Cook meat thoroughly: Make sure ground meat, sausages and poultry are cooked through to the center. Juices should run clear after cooking.

Wash fresh produce: Wash leafy greens, vegetables and fruits before eating them, even if they are pre-packaged.

Keep food at a safe temperature: 40–140°F (5–60°C) is the ideal temperature for the growth of bacteria. Don't leave leftovers sitting at room temperature. Instead, put them right in the fridge.

There are a number of steps you can take to reduce your risk of food poisoning. Practice good hygiene, check use-by dates, wash fruits and vegetables before eating them and keep food out of the temperature danger zone of 40–140°F (5–60°C). Food poisoning is an illness caused by eating food contaminated with bacteria, viruses or toxins. It can result in a range of symptoms such as stomach cramps, diarrhea, vomiting and even death.

Poultry, seafood, deli meat, eggs, unpasteurized dairy, rice, fruits and vegetables carry a high risk of food poisoning, especially when they're not stored, prepared or cooked properly. To minimize your risk, follow the simple tips listed above to ensure you take special care when buying, handling and preparing these foods.

WHAT SUPPORTIVE THERAPIES TREAT FOOD POISONING?

Food poisoning can cause nausea and vomiting. These symptoms generally resolve on their own without medication, but there are some precautions you can take to avoid complications and ease discomfort. Food poisoning occurs when you ingest pathogens through food. This can result in gastroenteritis, which involves unpleasant symptoms like nausea, vomiting, and diarrhea. Depending on the pathogen, the symptoms of food poisoning usually pass on their own within a few days. However, it can be very unpleasant, and you risk becoming dehydrated.

Stay hydrated

Food poisoning can cause dehydration. Excessive vomiting and diarrhea can lead to your body expelling too much water. When too much water is lost, your body may have difficulty performing basic functions. To avoid severe dehydration, which needs to be treated in a hospital, try to stay hydrated at home. Sip water when possible. Use an electrolyte solution, which can be bought over the counter (OTC) at a pharmacy. If you don't have an electrolyte drink, you can make your own using:

1/2 teaspoon salt

6 teaspoons sugar

1 liter (4.2 cups) water

Be sure not to add more salt or sugar than specified, as this can be dangerous.

If you're not able to keep water down, or if you're unable to drink at all, it's important to seek medical attention. Severe dehydration is treated with intravenous fluids.

Sip ginger tea

If you're feeling up to it, try drinking ginger tea.

Not only is it a way to stay hydrated, but it may also relieve the symptoms of food poisoning. Some researchTrusted Source suggests that ginger could help relieve nausea and vomiting, although more clinical trials are needed to verify this.

Rest

It's important to avoid exerting yourself through physical activity because gastroenteritis puts you at risk for dehydration. Although the vomiting and diarrhea might last as little as a few hours, it might take longer for your energy levels to return to usual.

Try a warm compress

Gastroenteritis and food poisoning can cause abdominal discomfort. A warm compress, such as a microwavable beanbag or a hot water bottle, might bring you some relief.

Eat when possible

When you've stopped vomiting, try eating small portions of food. Rich food might irritate your stomach further, so you might prefer bland foods like:

crackers

bread

cereal

plain rice

bananas

Keep drinking fluids, too.

What OTC medications can help with food poisoning symptoms?

Your local pharmacist can suggest OTC medications for food poisoning.

Depending on your circumstances, you could get antidiarrheal medication such as loperamide (Imodium) or bismuth subsalicylate (Pepto-Bismol) to soothe diarrhea. A pharmacist might also suggest nonsteroidal anti-inflammatory drugs (NSAIDs) such as ibuprofen or naproxen. These medications can reduce stomach pain and fever. Additionally, it's a good idea to get electrolyte drinks or oral rehydration sachets, such as Pedialyte.

What clinical treatment options are available?

If vomiting and diarrhea don't resolve in a few hours, and if you cannot keep water down, it's best to go to the emergency room. Clinical treatment for food poisoning can include prescription medications, such as:

antiemetic (anti-vomiting) medication like chlorpromazine (Thorazine) and metoclopramide (Reglan and Metozolv)

antiparasitic medications such as metronidazole (Flagyl) or ivermectin (Stromectol) if you've been exposed to a parasite

To treat dehydration, you may be put on an IV drip. This replenishes your hydration levels intravenously.

When should you consult with a doctor or other healthcare professional?

Most of the time, you don't need to see a doctor or healthcare professional to recover from food poisoning. However, the Centers for Disease Control and Prevention (CDC)Trusted Source recommends seeking professional help if you:

have bloody diarrhea

have a fever over 102°F (39°C)

are unable to keep liquids down

have signs of dehydration, such as dizziness, little or no urination, and a very dry mouth and throat

experience diarrhea for more than 3 days

For children, especially babies, it's important to go to the emergency room if they can't keep liquids down.

Other frequently asked questions

What are the symptoms of food poisoning and other foodborne illnesses?

The symptoms of food poisoning can include:

diarrhea

fever

nausea

stomach cramps

vomiting

These symptoms commonly resolve in a day or two, but they might last longer depending on the pathogen that caused the poisoning.

What should you do if you suspect you have a foodborne illness?

You can usually recover from food poisoning and foodborne illnesses at home. During the recovery period, drink plenty of fluids, including water and electrolyte drinks. Get enough rest and consider using ibuprofen for fever and cramps. However, you should go to the emergency room if you:

have diarrhea for more than 3 days

have bloody diarrhea

have a fever over 102°F (39°C)

vomit up liquids

You should also seek emergency help if you have signs of dehydration, including:

dizziness

little or no urination

very dry mouth and throat

The CDC asks that you contact your local health departmentTrusted Source if you have or suspect you may have a foodborne illness.

How long does food poisoning last?

Food poisoning typically lasts a few days, but it can last weeks, depending on which pathogen caused food poisoning. For example:

Bacillus cereus, a form of bacteria, can cause symptoms that last 24 to 48 hoursTrusted Source.

Cryptosporidium causes symptoms that can last 1 to 2 weeksTrusted Source.

E. coli symptoms usually last 3 to 7 days.

Giardia lamblia symptoms can last 1 to 3 weeksTrusted Source.

Listeria symptoms can last 1 to 3 daysTrusted Source.

Norovirus symptoms usually last 1 to 3 days.

Rotavirus symptoms usually last 3 to 8 daysTrusted Source.

Salmonella symptoms can last 4 to 7 daysTrusted Source.

Contact emergency medical services if you experience diarrhea symptoms that last for more than 3 days or if your stools are bloody.

Can antibiotics treat food poisoning?

Yes, if the food poisoning was caused by bacteria. However, food poisoning can also be caused by viruses, so antibiotics won't work.

What can you do to prevent food poisoning?

To avoid food being contaminated by pathogens, practice good hygiene when preparing and eating food. For example:

Wash all food and cooking equipment before using it. Make sure you wash your hands before working with food or eating.

Keep foods refrigerated. Your refrigerator should be at 40°F (4°C) or below. Refrigerate fresh foods as soon as you get home from grocery shopping. The CDCTrusted Source recommends refrigerating leftovers within 2 hours of cooking.

Keep raw meat, poultry, eggs, and seafood away from other foods. Don't store them in the same container. Use separate cutting boards for raw meats.

Cook meat, seafood, eggs, and poultry at the right temperature to kill bacteria.

Discard food that has been left out for too long.

Avoid drinking contaminated water. When hiking, camping, or traveling to unfamiliar regions, be sure to check that the water you're drinking is safe.

Keep your eye on the FoodSafety.gov site to stay in the loop on product recalls and outbreaks of foodborne illnesses.

Food poisoning symptoms usually go away after a few days. While treating food poisoning at home, try to stay hydrated by drinking a lot of liquids, including electrolyte drinks.

You can also ease discomfort by resting and using a warm compress on your stomach. Some over-the-counter medications may provide relief.

WHY COOKING CHICKEN TO 165 DEGREES IS CRITICAL FOR ENSURING SAFETY, PREVENTING ILLNESS

In the study, researchers surveyed 3,969 households across five European countries about common methods for checking for chicken's doneness. They found there are a number of inadequate indicators of food safety. Using the chicken's meat or juice color to assess readiness is one such example. Although a popular method, researchers reported that the inner color of chicken changes at temperatures too low to kill common poultry pathogens such as Salmonella and Campylobacter.

Safely cooked poultry can vary in color from white to pink to tan, according to the United States Department of

Agriculture (USDA). The study's researchers also reported bacteria remaining on a chicken's surface even after cooking, suggesting alternative or additional methods of measuring safety are necessary. While thermometers can help, the researchers reported that only 1 in 75 households use them while cooking chicken.

Risks associated with raw chicken

Eating undercooked chicken causes foodborne illness resulting in high fever, digestive malfunction, and dehydration for more than 1 million people in the United States every year, according to the Centers for Disease Control and Prevention (CDC). The most common bacteria found in contaminated chicken is Campylobacter, but chicken may also contain Salmonella and Clostridium perfringensTrusted Source, says Caroline West Passerrello, MS, RDN, LDN, a spokesperson for the Academy of Nutrition and Dietetics. This is what she says people can expect after being infected by common chicken bacteria:

Most people who get ill from Salmonella can have diarrhea, fever, and stomach cramps that begin between 6 hours and 6 days after infection. Symptoms can last from 4 to 7 days.

People with Campylobacter infection experience similar symptoms starting 2 to 5 days after infection and lasting up to a week. Nausea and vomiting may also occur.

With C. perfringens, people develop diarrhea and abdominal cramps within 6 to 24 hours, typically 8 to 12 hours. The illness usually begins suddenly and lasts for less than 24 hours, but vomiting and fever aren't associated symptoms.

Safety starts at the grocery store

Experts agree that cooking chicken to at least an internal temperature of 165°F (74°C) is a better measure of food safety than any clock timer. But contamination and infection can occur before anyone eats the chicken. "Proper prep begins at the point of purchase.

CONCLUSION

Food poisoning can be caused by toxins or microorganisms in food or drinks. Symptoms may include vomiting, diarrhea, fever, and more.Food poisoning is extremely common, affecting an estimated 9.4 million Americans yearly. Food poisoning can be caused by bacteria-contaminated foods or by eating foods containing poisonous toxins, such as certain mushroom species. Symptoms and severity vary, and it could take hours to days for them to appear making identifying the offending food quite difficult.High risk foods include undercooked meat/chicken, eggs, unpasteurized dairy products, shellfish, and unwashed fruits/veggies.